INSTANT
EYESIGHT

Instant Eyesight

The INSTANT-Series *Presents*

INSTANT

EYESIGHT

How to Improve Eyesight Instantly!

Instant Series Publication

ISBN 978-1-515-33714-0

Printed in the United States of America

First Edition

FIRST STEP:

Before proceeding, visit http://www.instantseries.com, and join the **INSTANT Newsletter** now.

You will want to! :)

CONTENTS

Chapter 8: See Better for Tomorrow

Instant Eyesight

<u>Chapter 1</u>

Possible to Retrain Your Eyes?

The Magnificent Eyes

The **eyes** are complicated and delicate body parts. They help us sustain ourselves by providing key information about the environment around us. For this reason it is important to take care of your eyes with exercises and awareness.

In other words, in the same way that you might dedicate yourself to exercising and staying fit, you should also dedicate yourself to taking care of your eyes.

Take some time right now to think about the common experience of humanity these days. We spend an incredible amount of time in front of our computers, phones and other screens. Do we even enjoy the simple things in life anymore? The natural color of leaves, the hustle and bustle of the city block?

Nowadays there is little time to enjoy things away from our iPhones and computers. Not only do we *lose enjoyment of life* this way, we are steadily loosing the agility of our vision.

The Causes For Decline Of Vision

While some people suffer from **bad vision** starting in childhood, others won't develop real problems until later in life. These problems may be corrected to a certain degree by glasses and contact lenses, but the main issue is that people are still addicted to unhealthy habits that cause their problems to worsen.

The use of screens these days leads people to use their eye muscles less and less. They are using their brains first to process new information, which is then transferred to the eye. Normally this process would be done the other way around. The eye should be the one transmitting information to your brain. Do you understand the difference in this chain reaction?

Studies show that if you look back **20 years ago,** people would develop eyesight problems less frequently than nowadays and that our sight is degrading prematurely. These are the consequences of spending so much time on our phones and computers.

Treat Your Eyes Like Muscles

The <u>main idea</u> here is to help you reconnect you to your natural sight sensation by reducing your reliance on glasses or contact lenses. *Eye training exercises* are essential in these cases.

We can't predicate how our lives will go. Sometimes we are victims of improbable events such as breaking our glasses, forgetting them at home, or a contact lens falling out and getting lost. Maybe you wake up in the middle in the night having to go to the bathroom and you can't find your glasses. In those instances, *what do you do*?

In order to navigate your world under such circumstances it is important to **train your eyes** to function naturally, without glasses or lenses, for short periods of time.

Training your eyes can help with so many things!

1. **Eye focus.** Eye training exercises can help you improve your sight, especially if you suffer from double vision.

2. Paying attention to **details**. You will be more aware of the world around you.

3. **Adaptation.** You will be able to adapt and react to unexpected situations quickly, even in low or dark lighting.

4. **Fast recovery** from eye muscle pain that occurs after longer periods in front of a TV or computer screen.

The Inconvenience Of The Crutches

Here's an example where eye muscle training could come in handy...

Imagine that you are woken up late at night by a storm and realize that there's no more electricity. Since you can't see clearly in the dark, you have a hard time finding your glasses. You want to find the interrupter and try to switch the electricity back on, but you are so used to using your glasses, that you feel incapable of venturing into the dark without them.

You might as well be in a horror movie with a hideous monster waiting in the dark to get you!

You have to do something, because it's summer and without the A/C you are burning up. You won't be able to sleep like this. But what can you do when you can hardly see?

Perhaps if you knew how to **condition your eyes** to a low light environment you could have solved your problem easily!

Since we never know what comes ahead in life, it's best to be prepared. Glasses help you with your sight and are important for everyday life, but what can you do when the unexpected happens?

That's why eye exercise and training is so *important*! Continue on for exercises that you can do every day to improve your eyesight and train your eyes for the unexpected.

<u>Exercise</u>: Image Reproduction

Take a look at <u>Fig.1-5</u>.

Fig.1-5

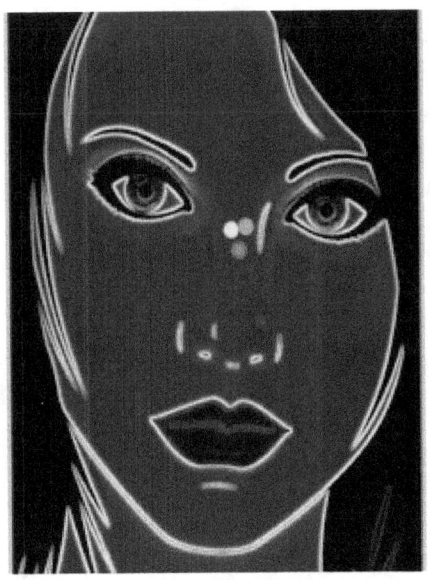

1.) Without the help of any eye accessory (glasses or lenses), look at the yellow, green, and red dots all at the same time.

2.) Look at them, without blinking, for **20 seconds**.

3.) After you've finished counting to 20, look at the wall in front of you.

4.) Write down what you see.

You should actually have the reflection of the image on your wall*!

This exercise is to help you realize that your eyes don't necessarily need glasses or lenses to be able to see beautiful colors, shapes, and images like this illustration. This simple and basic exercise just shows you how powerful eye focus can be.

Disclaimer

*Caution: Although eye training to improve your eyesight is encouraged, you shouldn't abandon your glasses or lenses completely, even if you feel that these training exercises are effective, especially while driving or working - NEVER put yourself at that kind of risk whenever you must have full accurate vision!

Not depending on eyewear all the time is a good thing, but remember, your eyesight will unfortunately fade as you get older and will probably not be fully restored.

<u>We recommend</u> that you still use your glasses or contact lenses in your everyday life. The proposed exercises, will help you use your eyes naturally when the necessity arises, but will not fully cure you from any vision impairments or eye diseases.

Always continue regular checkups with an optometrist.

Chapter 2

Develop Sharper Vision

A Double Vision Problem

Whether you have a hard time seeing what's ahead of you because you've left your glasses at home or you suffer from diplopia, where you see everything as double, the outcome is the same.

The inability to know your surroundings can be incredibly frustrating and confusing. Seeing obstacles or common objects in **double** (like an electricity pole ahead of you for instance) can cause many problems, not the least of which is choose the wrong image to run through.

You can spend minutes, sometimes, straining your eye muscles, trying to focus your vision on an object, but it just won't work. You only end up putting too much effort on a dysfunctional eye nerve, sometimes causing *terrible headaches*. This make you depend even more on glasses or contact lenses.

The following is an exercise that will directly help you learn to be less dependent on your glasses and instead be able to rely on your natural eyesight when necessary.

<u>Exercise</u>: Eye Pushups

This eye exercise can be done anywhere. On your commute to work, in your office, or waiting on your fast food order. You can be standing or seated. You just need your eyes!

<u>Follow these steps:</u>

1.) Take your glasses off and find an **elongated object** like a pen, pencil, or a bottle (preferably empty).

2.) *Mark your object* or find a noticeable marking (like a letter or picture) already on it.

3.) Start bringing the object close to your eyes (both eyes should be focused on the marking).

4.) Make an effort *not to blink* and put all your attention and focus on the marking.

5.) When the item is very close to your eyes (just a little away from your nose) **stop.** Keep your eyes on the mark.

6.) Bring the item back a few inches away from your eyes, still focusing on the mark.

7.) Repeat this, moving the object back and forth about **7 or 10 times.**

8.) If somehow you still see double after the object is brought closer to your eyes, stop and restart the process by bringing the object away, and starting from the beginning.

<u>Answer these questions</u> after completing the exercise:

- How many times did you have **double vision** after moving the object closer to your face?

- Could you feel the pulsing sensation on your eye muscles during and after completing the exercise? Explain this sensation.

- How focused was your vision right after your first training with this technique?

How Eye Pushups Help In Real Life

Eye pushups not only let the eye muscles get used to this effort instantly, but they also facilitate the <u>blood flow</u> in the area around your eyes so that you can actually feel the blood pumping through the veins around your eyes.

This is an indication that your eye muscles are working, and is hopefully something you will notice the very first time you do this exercise. If you do eye pushups every day you will condition your eyes to make adjustments and focus quickly. The more you **practice** it, the more you'll start seeing improvements.

Eye pushups are good for people who have *crossed vision*, for those who see *double*, and those who wish to have a *focused vision* when trying to identify an object from afar.

You should be able to avoid poles in front of you, dog poop on the sidewalk, or even wild animals (you certainly don't want your double vision to confuse a wild bear with a bush).

Eye pushups are applicable to everyday occurrences.

- **Useful Tip**: If your double vision occurs all of a sudden, find a fixing point on the object in front of you. Imagine a dot, or the same marking you are used to when you do your exercises. *Focus your vision* on that marking as you approach it. It will result in you having a clearer vision of what's ahead of you and avoiding all sorts of trouble and accidents.

<u>Chapter 3</u>

Increase Distance of Eyesight

The Eye Of A Camera

Another way to improve vision problems is training the eye muscles to make your pupil enlarge in order to zoom in on whatever is your focal points. This time, you will not only work with your eyes, but with your brain too!

This exercise is good for people with <u>blurred vision</u> or a <u>lazy eye.</u>

Imagine that your face was dotted with a mechanical engine inside your head. You can actually activate this engine by turning a lever manually to the right that would enable you to zoom in on images, and then to the left in order to zoom out from those same images. (See it as how a camera works when you want to capture more details in a photograph.)

It's very complicated to achieve this technique because you have to **coordinate** your eyes with your brain.

<u>Exercise</u>: Zoom In. Zoom Out.

Let's try it! <u>Follow these steps:</u>

1.) Find a space that is crowded with many objects where you can practice this technique, like your garden, a park or a messy office.

2.) Capture a view of this space in your mind by fixing your attention on it for **1-2 minutes**.

3.) *Memorize several details* about your environment in turn.

4.) Visualize these details by citing them and having them appear in your head first (you can keep your eyes open here, you just have to maintain a good level of concentration).

5.) Try to **enhance** the image in your brain.

6.) Go through the small details and mentally **zoom in** on them each of them.

7.) Make a projection of these details by *opening your eyes* as wide as possible. Even though the objects are not moving they will seem bigger, as if they are right in front of you.

8.) The **zooming out** occurs as soon as you relax the eyes so they aren't open as wide.

The eye serves as a transmitter of information (images) to the brain. The brain processes these images and helps you identify them.

Heightened Sensory Vision

What is interesting about this technique of zooming in and out on your surroundings, is that it helps you appreciate the scenery around you when blurred vision or lazy eye might have prevented you.

Through this technique you learn to *pay more attention* to detail, naturally—as if you had perfect eyesight. You can admire unknown environments without being lost or trying to interpret it solely with your brain.

Here, we can say that your eyes, play **almost 70%** of the work by trying to transfer as much information to the brain, which in turn only helps you go through the information and then retransmits it to the eye. You eye muscles are stimulated and working very fast and effectively, without the need of your glasses or technology like Google Maps.

No Need To Strain To See Farther

If you have blurry vision when you try to focus your eyes on an object, you can suffer from eye muscle strain. This strain can cause unbearable pain to your optic nerves and even uncontrollable teary eyes. Under such circumstance you might opt to forgo looking at the world around you and instead look at pictures on your phone.

This **zooming technique**, however, will help <u>train your muscles</u> to focus your eyes more easily without straining.

This technique is especially interesting, as it gets you to enjoy and discover scenery with intense sensation. Your eyes will almost work like a **touch screen**—allowing you to optimize the size of an image by clicking on it and enlarging it with your fingers.

Everyone should enjoy discovering textures, shapes and art with their own eyes. Now, with the use of this technique you can do just that and your optical muscles won't need to strain themselves.

Chapter 4

Distinguish Objects Better

Mistaken Distinction

It can be frustrating sometimes when you try to grab something and then accidentally grab something else that was close to it. Some of the time, you don't even realize you've grabbed the wrong thing.

Maybe, *for example*, instead of your car keys, you grab your wife's bangle bracelets. You might not even realize until you try to open up your car and in your hand all you see are those bracelets.

The problem here consists of having difficult time differentiating objects that are side by side, especially without your eyewear. This type of eye impairment might not seem crucial, but it should be taken seriously, as it can worsen with time or even put you in danger.

Imagine that you are trying to get some pain medication from your medicine cabinet, and instead you pick some other pills that have diuretic effects and by the time you decide to verify the package and read the instructions you are stuck to the toilet! *Yikes!*

Many people would go see an optometrist right away to try and correct this problem, but there's a *natural way* to correct this anomaly and help you have a better visual focus every time.

<u>Exercise</u>: Test Your Visual Focus

This exercise will help you to transfer the right information to your brain, so that it can do its role by *coordinating the movements* of your hands with your eyes (when you want to grab your keys, your hands should be guided by your eyes to grab those keys). It seems so simple, but can feel impossible sometimes.

Let's follow along here:

1.) Choose a specific object and place it in an area **surrounded** by many other objects, maybe of similar shape and size.

2.) Remove your glasses or contact lenses.

3.) Maintain your focus solely on the one object from a short distance, without blinking or looking elsewhere for **at least a minute**. If this puts too much pressure on your eyes or they start tearing up—don't worry, it simply means that your optical muscles are at work. With practice your eyes won't tear up as much.

4.) Move closer to the object to accomplish total concentration and focus on it again for **about a minute**.

5.) Finally, back away from the object, still focusing on it with your eyes.

6.) <u>Repeat</u> the exercise at least **3 times**.

Now, answer the following questions:

- Did you notice an increase in focus when attempting the exercise a second time? Explain.

- How soon, did you notice you weren't experimenting "the teary eye" effect? Explain.

Your brain and eyes are conditioned to *work together*. The purpose of this exercise is to train your optical muscles to build up some strength and endurance each time you have your eyes on a single item.

Strengthen The Bond Between Eye And Brain

Eye and brain miscommunication (commonly diagnosed as amblyopia) doesn't only happen when you want to grab an object, it also happens when you try to read.

It sometimes happens that you see another word in place of the actual word written in the text. It's a common symptom for those diagnosed with "lazy eye," where the brain automatically deciphers a word as a totally different one.

For this type of inconvenient optical problem, you can still use this focus training in order to strengthen your eye muscles and reduce the chance of your brain tricking you.

Chapter 5

Exercise Your Eyes

Eye Workouts

Our next two **eye exercises** (laser drawing and directional eye) should be relief if you have limited visual faculties and just want to enjoy your vision, without the burden of the glasses.

For instance, if you have a hard time, staring at an object for a certain amount of time (normally for more than a minute), there are options to solidify and strengthen your optical muscles. You will still use your eyes and a little bit of your eye muscles, but <u>head rotation</u> will also help you complete your eye training.

People with refractive visual errors caused by *blurred vision, glaucoma or strabismus* (also known as, crossed eyes), should practice these exercises constantly, as they will help them gain some improvement to their condition.

<u>Eye Exercise</u>: Laser Drawing

The first eye exercise, is quite fun and it is called **laser drawing exercise**. Just like its name indicates, pretend you have laser beams shooting out from your eyes that you can use to draw on the wall in front of you. (If you ever wish you were a superhero, now you can pretend.)

Draw something *very basic* that will actually lead you to move your eyes, eye muscles and neck (or head) around with ease. The basic shapes to draw would be numbers or letters. To keep it simple for this initial exercise, choose a **one digit number** between 0 and 9.

1.) Start with your head facing straight forward, preferably facing a blank wall.

2.) Begin drawing a number. We'll use the **number 6** as an example.

3.) Start with the top part of the number (always start with the "little tail" first or the left part of any other number that doesn't have a tail).

4.) <u>Follow the number's shape</u> all the way down, by moving your eyes and neck in the same direction, at the same time.

5.) Make sure, your eyes and your neck make the same movements, at the same time. The neck is used to avoid too much strain on the optical muscle.

6.) Now, go back up, and end up with the lower part of the number (the flattened circle). You are basically *drawing this number*, the same way you would do it if you were actually writing it down on a piece of paper.

7.) *Be very gentle*, and take smooth breaths in between movements.

Drawing these letters and numbers with your eyes, will help you "connect" with their shape and identify them easily. This means that even though you can't always see perfectly, or your brain sometimes has no coordination with your eyes, you will be able to **recognize** these common shapes readily.

In a sense you are learning to write, all over again. Instead of using your hands, and thus developing muscles in that area, you are *developing your eye muscles* with no strain on them because the neck movement supports them.

Widening Peripheral Range Of Vision

Trying to enjoy a great view, can be difficult for some. <u>Think about it.</u> You have to turn your head and eyes from left to right, up and down, at all times. Often times, people with poor eyesight caused by a lack of eye coordination or weak optical muscles end up with strong migraines or their eyes hurting by the end of the day.

This can be so painful, stressful, and a bit depressing, since it means that those suffering from these migraines have a lot of limitations to the fun that is out there. If you are one of them, you are certainly missing out on a lot!

Perhaps these repercussions of eye strain make you prefer to spend time surfing the web or playing a game on your phone with your glasses on, while others are cheering about some animals during a safari tour or enjoying the sights of the Niagara Falls.

Don't we all want to enjoy the simple things in life? You only live once, and your eye problems are keeping you away from a lot of things. Why not try to put those glasses down for a minute and **enjoy the beautiful sights,** by simply knowing how to strengthen your eyes effectively?

So, instead of having narrow vision or letting your eye muscles give up easily (aching because of the effort), train your eyes to move left and right. This will help your visual focus become wider, resulting in you being able to visualize many details at the same time.

Eye Exercise: Directional Eye

Let's now have a look at our next exercise simply called the **directional eye exercise.** It still has to do with developing eye muscles, but focuses on preparing your eyes to have a wider range of vision.

This is how it works:

- When you are confronted with a **complex image** (like for instance a painting or a breathtaking view in nature), you should first look from left to right, then bring your sight from the upper right to the bottom left and finally bring it to the right once more.

- If you are trying to watch **something in motion,** trace an imaginary black line, while you follow the object in motion with your eyes.

- When you are trying to watch something that is **moving towards you** (like a person, for instance), make the left to the right movement with your eyes to then bring your sight from the upper right to the bottom left and finally bring it to the right once more. Next, make an eye movement, going from the top of the object to the bottom, so that you can follow the object moving towards you with your eye. This can be done for objects situated from a certain distance from you, and for those situated a few inches away.

<u>Practicing</u> this should result in your eye muscles being trained to make the right movements, where instead of simply staring at an object, they move in many directions in a fraction of a second while strengthening themselves at the same time.

The technique will consist of you building up a "frame of vision" by moving your eyes from left to right, and then from the bottom right to the bottom left, and then to the right again, so as to cover as many details as possible about the scenery.

Let's now move on to practice all these exercises and theories right next to each other.

Chapter 6

Train Your Eye Muscle

Practice 1: Give Me 10 With Your Eyes!

1.) Pick a horizontal object (pencil, paper, bottom, etc.), and find or make a marking on it for your eyes to focus on.

2.) With that horizontal object in your hand, <u>stretch your hand</u> in front of you.

3.) Start fixing your vision on the marking (try not to blink).

4.) Move the object towards you, maintaining your focus on it. When the object is brought close enough to your eyes (almost touching the tip of your nose), **stop**!

5.) Maintain the same concentration. Keep your eyes on the marking for about **20 seconds**.

6.) Stretch your arm away again, still maintaining your eyes on the marking.

7.) Repeat this horizontal push up session **10 times**, each time you decide to do this exercise.

Practice 2: Draw With Your Eyes

Fig.6-2

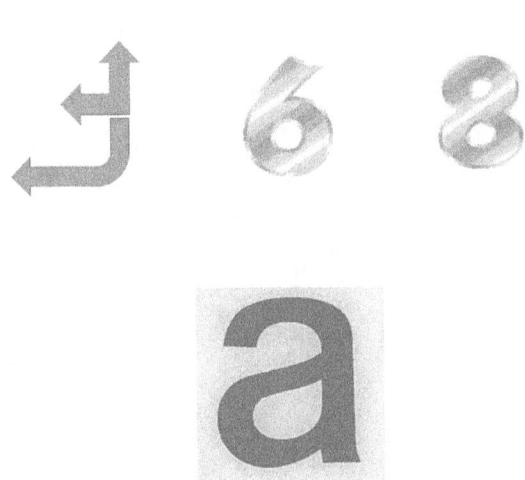

- Following the guidelines from the **laser drawing exercise**, reproduce the shape, numbers and letter, on the figure above.

Helpful Tip!: Remember, that laser drawing works exactly like writing with your hands, so if you are hesitating on where to start when using your eyes as a drawing tool, practice writing the shapes, numbers, and letters first and then follow the same pattern with your eyes.

<u>Practice 3</u>: Navigate With Your Eyes

Considering the **directional eye exercise,** how would you quickly cover the landscape on the figure below (<u>Fig.6-3</u>)?

Fig.6-3

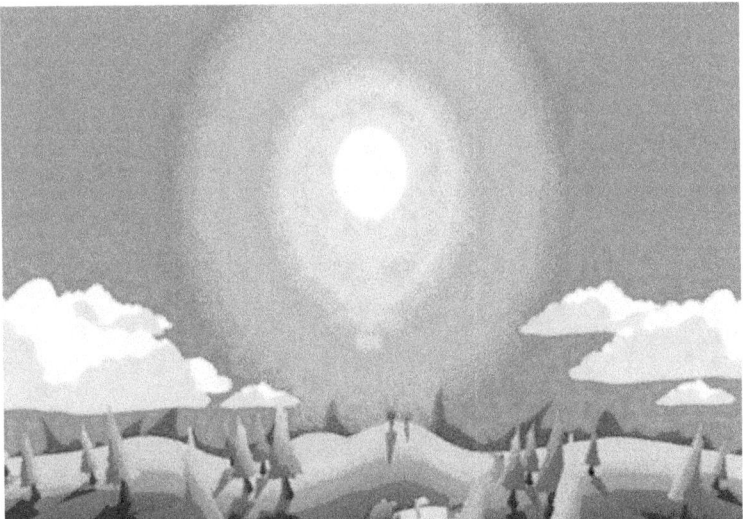

Will you need to draw an imaginary line or cover the image up and down with your eyes?

- <u>Justify your answer</u> by explaining how you should proceed when facing this type of view.

<u>Practice 4</u>: Identify At Long Distance With Your Eyes

Fig.6-4

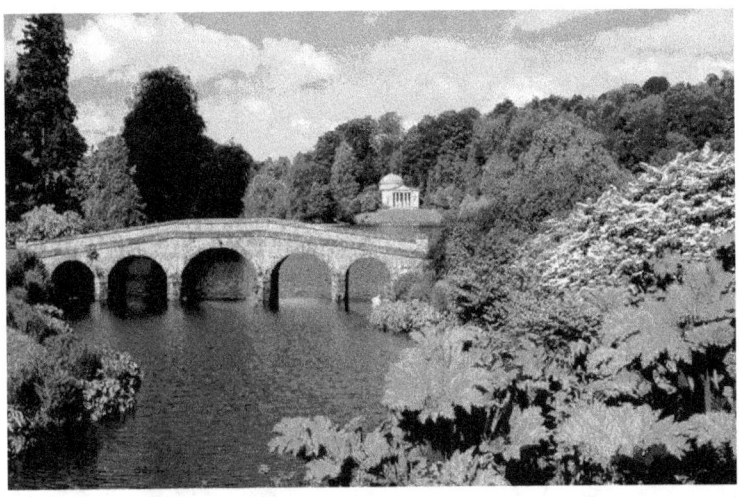

Take a look at this image (<u>Fig.6-4</u>). It's very lush and full of color and so many details; one must admit that this is a fantastic scene to witness.

If you suffered from a <u>lazy eye</u> or <u>blurred vision</u>, how would you proceed in identifying the building in the background?

- *Give a detailed explanation* of the technique that helps you enhance details that are far away.

Chapter 7

Incorporate Habits to Support Eyes

Other Things You Can Do For Your Eye Health

Natural sight improvement shouldn't rely solely on eye training exercises. There are other simple tips that make a lot of differences in how your muscles will react to light, new objects, movement, and other details during the day.

These habits might even be things you do normally over the course of your day.

For example, a lot of people like to rub their hands together and place their palms on their eyes, while others will massage their temples when they have a headache.

Generally, people feel that this helps "awaken" their senses or relieves tension in the mind and eyes.

Most of us don't realize it, but these gestures are <u>very beneficial</u> to our optic nerves, and help with blood circulation in the area around the eye.

<u>Habit 1</u>: Palming

<u>Palming</u> describes the act of rubbing your hands together so as to warm them up, and then gently placing them on your eyelids. The rubbing together of the hands should last for **at least 20 seconds** and then they should be kept on your eyes for **about 15 seconds.**

When you remove your hands and open your eyes you will see multicolored sparkles (think of it like a private fireworks show!) in front of you, like your eyes are waking up from a long sleep. Your eyes will feel a little heavy.

This condition has less to do with the little pressure you've put on them and more to do with the fact that your nerves and eye muscles are getting <u>warmed up</u>.

Palming can be a great warm up session to your eye training exercises or it can simply be a technique to use whenever your eyes need a little boost.

<u>Habit 2</u>: Gentle Massage

A **gentle rubbing** of your eye contour can do wonders! This is ideal for those having weak eye muscles or weak eye coordination.

Use your *index* and your *middle finger* and start making very gentle circular movements outside of the eye socket. From right-to-left on the left eye and from left-to-right on the right one.

Start from the area of the nose called the **tear trough** (the space between the eye and the nose bridge) and move up to the corners of the eyes to end up back at the tear trough again.

Look at these two habits as <u>reviving sessions</u> where your fingers and palms respectively work as electric shock tools to your optic nerves and muscles. They work like successful resuscitation attempts done at hospitals for patients who suddenly stop breathing. Nurses, in these situations, rush to grab the defibrillator and perform a cardiac massage so as to resuscitate the patient. Here the defibrillator can be seen as your fingers or palms, and the patient is your eye.

Both techniques help you revive your eye muscles and should be done constantly, they can be considered <u>habits</u> to adopt regularly, rather than <u>exercises</u>.

<u>Habit 3</u>: Healthy Eating

Recommendations for a healthy body wouldn't be complete if <u>nutrition</u> wasn't included. The eyes are no exception to this rule; they are one of the most important parts of our body. Our eyesight depends not only on how we use our optic muscles but also on *what we eat* every day.

There are lots of foods you can eat to improve your eyesight or prevent diseases that effect the eyes. We will focus on **6** of them that are very common and important to eye health.

From now on it would be a good idea to leave room in your diet for:

1. <u>Carrots</u>*: These are found in many dishes (stew, stir-fry, and salad) and are a very common vegetable. They contain a type of vitamin A, called beta-carotene, that helps the retina (a layer behind the eyeball, where visual images are formed) and other parts of the eye to function properly. You can *eat them raw* as a snack or *steamed* to preserve the most nutrients.

*Helpful Tip!: All *orange colored* fruits and veggies are known to promote eye health! Keep this in mind from now on when you go grocery shopping.

2. <u>Leafy Greens</u>: Kale, spinach, collard greens and lettuce are all very rich in Zeaxanthin (which is found around the retina) and Lutein. Both of these nutrients lower the risk of developing cataracts, an eye disease that can occur late in life.

3. <u>Eggs</u>: The **yolk of the egg** is said to contain a high source of Lutein, Zeaxanthin and Zinc, which help the reduce risks of macular degeneration (loss of vision) and cataracts. It is best to *boil your eggs* in order to keep as many nutrients as possible.

4. <u>Citrus & Berries</u>: You can eat delicious fruits, *fresh or dried* (notably "goji berry," which has been used in traditional Chinese medicine to promote healthy eyesight and is available at most health food stores), and they are a nice compliment to your breakfast cereal or yogurt parfait. They are rich in vitamin C which also plays a huge role in decreasing the risk of developing eye diseases and sight deficiencies in the long term.

5. _Almonds_: Commonly found in snack bars or part of cereal mixes found in grocery stores everywhere, **almonds** are not too hard to come by. They are rich in vitamin E and just a handful during the day will help you get enough vitamin E daily to promote healthy eyes.

6. _Fatty Fish_: Tuna, salmon, mackerel, anchovies and trout are **fatty fish** known to be very _rich in DHA_ (a fatty acid found in your eye, specifically in the retina). People who eat these types of fish are less prone to dry eye syndrome which can prevent your eyes from providing enough moisture. Very uncomfortable!

Eating healthy to promote or improve good eyesight isn't that hard, huh? You can still eat food that is tasty and nutritious anytime, anywhere and you don't have too spend much either.

Simple habits such as palming and massaging your eyes don't demand too much of your time or large amounts of space. Furthermore, eating food to promote good eye health is *accessible, affordable, and delicious.*

Chapter 8

See Better for Tomorrow

Free Your Eyes

Our eyewear is such an important accessory. If you lose your glasses or lenses you can feel almost blind and helpless. There is really no need to remind you that you use them to read, see the world, and avoid any unnecessary burden put on your optic muscles, which can lead to aggravation and headaches for some.

This is understandable. But what happens when you lose your glasses/contacts or want to experience seeing the world naturally again, through the eyes you were born with? Shouldn't you be prepared?

While some of us are born with eyesight disabilities, with the *advanced research nowadays*, it is possible to isolate the role of the optic nerves and muscles in order to improve your vision.

Even in the worst case of eye disease, you can improve your eyesight <u>overnight</u> by simply strengthening those muscles, knowing how to warm them up, or eating the right foods.

Care For Your Eyes

Like the rest of the human body, optic muscles need training and care and as surprising as it might sound, you can do a few "pushups" per day to condition them for a better performance.

Having blurry vision can develop because of too much superficial lighting in your life. If you admire colors and the details of nature through your screen instead of witnessing them "live," maybe it's time to think about a change to your lifestyle.

Always warm up and strengthen those optic muscles whenever you can. Treat your eyes well, and you'll see a difference in your lifestyle that could change the rest of your life.

Instant Eyesight

An INSTANT Thank You!

Thank you for entrusting in the <u>INSTANT Series</u> to help you improve your life.

Our goal is simple, help you achieve instant results as fast as possible in the quickest amount of time. We hope we have done our job, and you have gotten a ton of value.

If you are in any way, shape, or form, dissatisfied, then please we encourage you to get refunded for your purchase because we only want our readers to be happy.

If, *on the other hand*, you've enjoyed it, if you can kindly leave us a review on where you have purchased this book, that would mean a lot.

What is there to do now?

Simple! Head over to http://www.instantseries.com, and sign up for our **newsletter** to stay up-to-date with the latest instant developments *(if you haven't done so already).*

Be sure to check other books in the INSTANT Series. If there is something you like to be added, be sure to let us know for as always we love your feedback.

Yes, we're on **social medias.** *Don't forget to follow us!*

https://www.facebook.com/InstantSeries

https://twitter.com/InstantSeries

https://plus.google.com/+Instantseries

Thank you, and wish you all the best!
- *The INSTANT Series Team*

Instant Eyesight

www.ingramcontent.com/pod-product-compliance
Lightning Source LLC
Chambersburg PA
CBHW070351300526
45791CB00025B/2025